NISTIR 7497

Security Architecture Design Process for Health Information Exchanges (HIEs)

Matthew Scholl
Kevin Stine
Computer Security Division
Information Technology Laboratory
National Institute of Standards and Technology
Gaithersburg, MD 20899

Kenneth Lin
Daniel Steinberg
Booz Allen Hamilton

September 2010

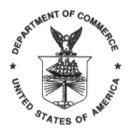

U.S. Department of Commerce
Gary Locke, Secretary

National Institute of Standards and Technology
Patrick D. Gallagher, Director

Acknowledgements

The authors, Matthew Scholl and Kevin Stine from NIST and Kenneth Lin and Daniel Steinberg from Booz Allen, wish to thank their colleagues and reviewers who contributed greatly to the document's development. A special note of thanks goes to Denise Tauriello and Christina Salameh from Booz Allen for their keen and insightful assistance throughout the development of this document. The authors also gratefully acknowledge and appreciate the many contributions from individuals in the public and private sectors whose thoughtful and constructive comments improved the quality and usefulness of this publication.

TABLE OF CONTENTS

TABLES AND FIGURES

1.0   Executive Summary

Protecting electronic patient health information is crucial to developing systems and structures that support the exchange of that information among healthcare providers, payers, and consumers using Health Information Exchanges (HIEs).[1] As noted in the Summary of the Nationwide Health Information Network (NHIN) report from the Office of the National Coordinator, "An important core competency of the HIE is to maintain a trusting and supportive relationship with the organizations that provide data to, and retrieve data from, one another through the HIE. The trust requirement is met through a combination of legal agreements, advocacy, and technology for ensuring meaningful information interchange in a way that has appropriate protections."[2]

The purpose of this publication is to provide a systematic approach to designing a technical security architecture for the exchange of health information that leverages common government and commercial practices and that demonstrates how these practices can be applied to the development of HIEs. This publication assists organizations in ensuring that data protection is adequately addressed throughout the system development life cycle, and that these data protection mechanisms are applied when the organization develops technologies that enable the exchange of health information.

This operating model will help organizations that are implementing HIEs to:

- Understand major regulations and business drivers;
- Identify cross-organizational enabling services;
- Define supporting business processes (for each service);
- Develop notional architectures (as a blueprint to support services, processes, and the selection of technical solutions); and
- Select technical solutions.

2.0   Introduction

The secure exchange of electronic health information is important to the development of electronic health records (EHRs) and to the improvement of the U.S. healthcare system. While the U.S. healthcare system is widely recognized as one of the most clinically advanced in the world, costs continue to rise, and often preventable medical errors occur. Health information technology (HIT), especially the development of electronic health records for use in both inpatient and ambulatory care settings, has the potential for providing reliable access to health information and thereby improving the healthcare system. However, the prospect of storing, moving, and sharing health information in electronic formats raises new challenges on how to ensure that the data is adequately protected.

---

[1] For the purpose of this document, HIE refers to an entity consisting of several organizations within a region or community sharing health information electronically, whereas "the exchange of health information" refers to the activity of transmitting health information among HIE component organizations. The security architecture design process will be of value in conducting the exchange of health information in general, as well as when initiating and establishing an HIE.

[2] Summary of the NHIN Prototype Architecture Contracts, A Report for the Office of the National Coordinator for Health IT, 31 May 2007.

Currently, health information[3] is scattered among various parties, including providers and payers, with patients maintaining limited control over the collection, access, use, and disclosure of their health information. The challenge of protecting this health information is exacerbated when an electronic version of health information can be shared much more easily than health records are exchanged today. The protection of patients' health information is an important factor in the adoption of the EHR.

Integrating security across different business and technical layers is necessary in order to address complex data protection challenges for the exchange of health information and HIEs. This publication presents a five-layered architecture design process as a systematic approach to identify and implement security and privacy. The five layers, or phases of activity, required for ensuring the protection of this form of data are: 1) capstone policies; 2) enabling services; 3) enabling processes; 4) notional architectures; and 5) technology solutions and standards. The security architecture design process provides a scalable, standardized, and repeatable methodology to guide HIE system development in the integration of data protection mechanisms across each layer, and results in a technology selection and design that satisfies high-level requirements and mitigates identified risks to organizational risk tolerances.

2.1 Purpose and Scope

The purpose of this publication is to provide a systematic approach to designing a technical security architecture for the exchange of health information by leveraging common government and commercial practices, and to demonstrate how these practices can be applied to the development of HIEs. The publication defines the five layers of this design process, their purposes and their relationships, and how they work together to facilitate the secure exchange of health information.

To exchange health information, two or more organizations will be involved. To secure the exchange of health information, the exchanging organizations and the means of conducting the exchange must have appropriate security and privacy controls. This publication focuses specifically on the exchange of health information and assumes that the exchanging organizations have an established security architecture to protect health information before and after the exchange. To ensure that health information is adequately protected, the "non-exchange" portions of the data usage, including collection, storage, modification, and destruction, must also receive security and privacy protections, which may include contingency and disaster recovery planning, configuration management, and other processes and technologies. This publication acknowledges the importance of those protections, but does not discuss the development of the entire information technology architecture of an HIE.

Many organizations must comply with data protection laws at the federal, state, and local levels that require them to conduct certain activities under specific operational parameters. While this publication does not directly address nontechnical issues such as those related to laws, regulations, and policies, specific roles and responsibilities, training, human resources issues, or nontechnical privacy issues, it does describe an architecture design process that allows for their integration into the information technology architecture of an HIE.

---

[3] This document uses the term "health information" as it is suitably broad and well-understood by the health information technology community. While the term is defined and used by the HIPAA Security and Privacy Rules, note that the material in this document may also be instructive to healthcare entities that are not HIPAA-covered entities, and to the development of systems that will contain health information that is not also protected health information (PHI) as defined by the HIPAA Rules.

The security architecture process applies to the exchange of health information and the deployment of HIEs. The architecture can be used to protect health information at various risk and sensitivity levels. This process, for example, can accommodate high-risk health information, such as information about treatments provided to particular patients, as well as lower-risk information, such as information that may be publicly available through other means yet remains sensitive in combination.

This document does not address governance or legal issues. HIEs should consult with legal counsel to identify applicable laws and regulations that will impact their operations and infrastructures, as well as to develop other legal documents such as memoranda of understanding (MOUs), contracts, data use and reciprocal support agreements, and service-level agreements (SLAs).

While the main focus of this document is security architecture, it is understood that privacy protections are essential to the collection, access, use, and disclosure of health information. For the purposes of this document, technical assurance of privacy is viewed as a subset of confidentiality. Implementation of security technologies that support confidentiality objectives may in turn support the technical implementation of privacy policy.

2.2 Audience

The principal audience for this publication includes HIE executives, HIE security policy developers, HIE security architects, and technical solution providers. These individuals will be most interested in its objective of providing an approach to developing the security architecture necessary for an HIE. These groups may be involved in different stages of the HIE life cycle. This document considers all stages of that life cycle, and can therefore assist each of the aforementioned groups in identifying appropriate technologies for HIEs under development, or in evaluating the effectiveness and appropriateness of technologies already in use in existing HIEs.

2.3 Document Organization

The remaining sections of this document discuss the following:

- Section 3.0, *HIE Contexts*, describes the scope and characteristics of the four main HIE contexts discussed in this document.

- Section 4.0, *HIT Security Architecture Design Process*, introduces the five-layer operating model that can be used for designing a security architecture to support the exchange of health information.

- Section 5.0, *Capstone Policies – Layer 1*, identifies and describes many major U.S. laws, regulations, and guidelines that influence and, in many cases, drive the development of an organization's unified policies ("Capstone Policies") for ensuring the secure exchange of health information.

- Section 6.0, *Enabling Services – Layer 2*, identifies and discusses twelve services, derived from common industry-wide practices, necessary to implement organizations' Capstone Policies.

- Section 7.0, *Enabling Processes – Layer 3*, describes processes that expand the Enabling Services into detailed, HIE-specific business requirements.

- Section 8.0, *Notional Architecture – Layer 4*, identifies architecture design principles and constructs that will serve as inputs, along with Capstone Policies and Enabling Services and Processes, to create a Notional Architecture, which is a blueprint for developing and implementing technical solutions.

- Section 9.0, *Technology Solutions and Standards – Layer 5*, illustrates the steps to select the technical solutions and data standards that will satisfy the requirements specified in the Notional Architecture.

- Section 10.0, *Building a Nationwide HIE using Regional HIEs*, discusses using a federation of Regional HIEs to construct a Nationwide HIE with federated security services.

- Appendix A, *Applying the Security Architecture Design Process*, employs the five-layer design process to a specific American Health Information Community (AHIC[4]) Use Case to illustrate the analyses and considerations that need to be made when applying this model to the exchange of health information.

- Appendix B, *Acronyms*, identifies and defines acronyms used in this document.

- Appendix C, *Glossary*, defines terms used in this document.

- Appendix D, *References*, provides references and related source material.

3.0   HIE Contexts

There are many conditions under which health information can be exchanged. Information can be sent to and from many different kinds of entities, in various forms of media, and can be subject to a wide range of laws, regulations, and policies. The set conditions under which the information is transmitted is sometimes called the "context" of the information exchange. This section presents the four main HIE contexts - Ad Hoc, Regional, Multi-Regional, and Nationwide - for which this security architecture design process applies. Figure 1 illustrates the HIE contexts.

---

[4] The AHIC was a federally chartered advisory body assembled to make recommendations to the Secretary of the U.S. Department of Health and Human Services on how to accelerate the development and adoption of health information technology. It was disbanded in 2008. A successor group, the National eHealth Collaborative (NeHC), was established through a grant from the Office of the National Coordinator for Health IT to build on the AHIC's accomplishments. See http://www.nationalehealth.org/AboutUs/.

Figure 1. HIE Contexts

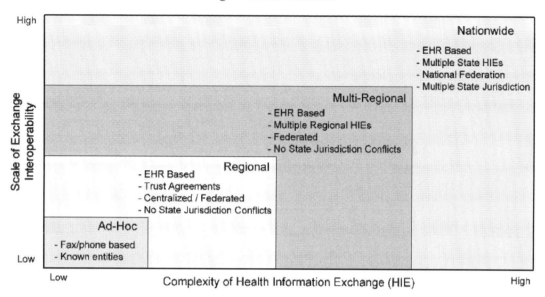

3.1 Ad Hoc HIEs

An Ad Hoc HIE occurs when two healthcare organizations exchange health information, usually under the precondition of familiarity and trust, using existing and usual office infrastructure such as mail, fax, e-mail, and phone calls. Health organizations that currently participate in Ad Hoc HIEs may find it impractical to justify the cost of migrating these activities into electronic health record (EHR)-based HIEs unless there are specific incentives making the process more appealing, or regional resources making the process easier. An Ad Hoc HIE can be effective for small-scale exchanges of health information, but Ad Hoc HIEs may not be able to integrate easily with each other in order to grow and expand. Such growth, or "scaling," requires familiarity with the participants and technologies used to create the infrastructure. Otherwise, the members of the Ad Hoc HIE may not have sufficient trust in the larger HIE and its participants to risk the privacy and security of their own information and systems.

3.2 Regional HIEs

Regional HIEs are those that consist of two or more legally and commercially independent institutions that share EHRs, but where no state jurisdictional issues exist that prevent or impede the sharing of data.[5] The HIE network includes clinicians, hospitals, labs, pharmacies, insurance companies, and other key health domain players. Participating organizations will normally draft a trust agreement to govern the information exchange. Depending on the scale, the technical architecture might be centralized or federated. Regional HIEs are large enough to justify the associated operational costs because the efficiencies realized offset these costs. They are simpler to administer than Multi-Regional and Nationwide HIEs because of their smaller scale and lack of state jurisdictional conflicts.

---

[5] Regional HIEs might include HIE members from different states. This document assumes that state jurisdiction conflicts, if any, have been reviewed and resolved.

3.3 Multi-Regional HIEs

Multi-Regional HIEs connect multiple Regional HIEs. They may cross state lines or other physical boundaries. They are usually EHR-based. Since they connect multiple Regional HIEs, they will likely have a federated technical architecture. For Multi-Regional HIEs, conflicts of laws may require complex solutions.

3.4 Nationwide HIEs

A Nationwide HIE would connect many Regional or Multi-Regional HIEs. It would require the use of some form of EHR, involve multiple state jurisdictions, and have a nationwide federated technical architecture. Multi-Regional and Nationwide HIEs have a different focus than Regional HIEs. Regional HIEs are basic building blocks that focus on developing effective and localized solutions to meet specific HIE needs (research, clinical trials, patient transfer, etc.). Multi-Regional and Nationwide HIEs focus on building the backbone infrastructure needed to connect various Regional HIEs.

This publication focuses on the needs of Regional HIEs. Assuming that the security architectures and other system aspects of Regional HIEs are interoperable, these HIEs can serve as the "building blocks" for larger Multi-Regional HIEs, and therefore represent a scalable solution for the ultimate emergence of a Nationwide HIE.

4.0   HIE Security Architecture Design Process

Technical solutions that facilitate the exchange of health information can be complex. With various policies and standards, and an ever-changing technical landscape, a systematic approach to designing an HIE security architecture can allow practitioners to analyze all policy requirements and ultimately refine them into a technology-neutral, vendor-neutral, standards-based architecture to drive technical solution decisions.

The use of a systematic approach plays a significant role in a successful and secure HIE implementation. The HIE security architecture design process was developed to assist HIEs in meeting this need by providing a five-layer methodology for successful HIE security technology identification and selection as illustrated in the following figure:

Figure 2. HIE Security Architecture Design Process

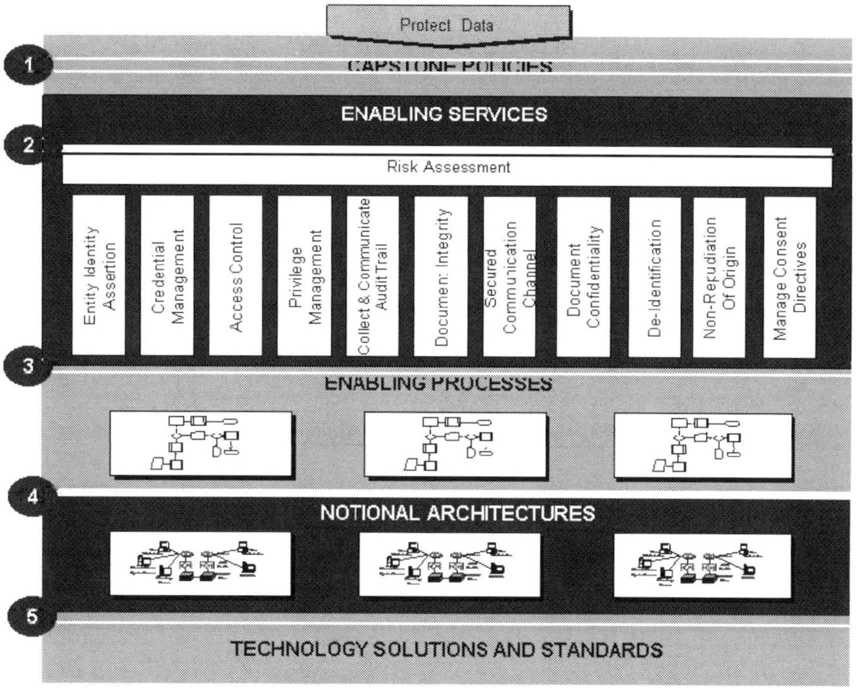

1) ***Capstone Policies:*** Capstone Policies are those developed by an organization that incorporates all requirements and guidance for protecting health information within HIEs. The contents and scope of Capstone Policies can be driven by state or federal laws or regulations, organizational policies, business needs, or policies developed for specific HIEs. The most efficient developer of the Capstone Policies will be the organization that can set standards for the entire HIE. A single participant in an HIE, for example, may be subject to a certain set of laws, but coordination across the entire HIE will be necessary to ensure that all drivers of Capstone Policies for all desired participants are identified and incorporated.

2) ***Enabling Services:*** Enabling Services define the nomenclature of services required to implement Capstone Policies. Enabling Services are designed to be HIE context-independent. Services presented in this publication are derived from common industry-wide data protection practices and then customized to specifically address the requirements of HIEs.

3) ***Enabling Processes:*** Enabling Processes define the operational baseline via use cases and scenarios for Enabling Services. Enabling Processes are HIE context-dependent. Two HIEs could, for example, have different Enabling Processes implementing the same Enabling Service (e.g., "Access Control").

4) ***Notional Architectures:*** Notional Architectures define the technical constructs (e.g., role-based access control and directory services) and their relationships to implement Enabling Processes. The Notional Architecture is the blueprint to drive the selection of technical solutions and data standards. The Notional Architecture is standards-based, technology-neutral, and vendor-neutral.

5) ***Technology Solutions and Standards:*** Technical solutions and data standards represent the selected technical solutions and data standards needed to implement the Notional Architecture.

Each layer of the design methodology is described in the following sections.

5.0   Capstone Policies – Layer 1

Capstone Policies are those policies that are developed by governing or coordinating institutions of HIEs. They provide overall requirements and guidance for protecting health information within and across those HIEs. Capstone Policies must address the requirements imposed by:

- all laws, regulations, and guidelines at the federal, state, and local levels;
- business needs; and
- policies at the institutional and HIE levels.

In developing Capstone Policies, organizations must identify the requirements that these laws, regulations, and other authorities impose on HIEs. One challenge in ascertaining that all such requirements have been identified is that these sources of requirements may not be specific to health information systems. For federally owned or operated systems, for example, other requirements such as the Federal Information Security Management Act (FISMA[6]) will also need to be considered. For this and other reasons, organizations must consider the expert input of appropriate legal counsel in assembling these requirements.

Within this section, many major U.S. federal laws relevant to the development of HIE security and privacy architectures are identified. For virtually all U.S. entities, however, other federal and state laws will also need to be considered. These representative laws are identified to illustrate the language, scope, and effects that such relevant laws may have. In particular, participants in a HIE will want to be aware of any relevant state laws in the course of developing their Capstone Policies. Under the Health Insurance Portability and Accountability Act (HIPAA), more stringent state laws that may require additional or greater protections for health information must be followed. The existence of HIPAA does not negate such requirements or excuse the covered entity from addressing them.

In many cases, relevant laws, regulations, and policies will impose other requirements aside from those that help identify Capstone Policies. These authorities may also establish broad goals or end states, without specifically defining Enabling Services, and may need to be interpreted based on industry best practices or reasonable safeguards. Addressing the text alone, therefore, may not be sufficient in order to ensure secure HIEs. In cases where authorities urge the institution of appropriate policies without proposing specific safeguards, practitioners should not confine themselves to developing Capstone Policies that merely satisfy compliance, but should view these authorities as setting only a minimum set of requirements. The HIPAA Security Rule, for example, explicitly encourages covered entities to develop security programs that are adequate, not merely to develop programs that nominally address the letter of the Rule. A covered entity's security program must be appropriate for its particular mission and goals. The preamble to the Security Rule notes that its standards "establish a minimum level of security to be met by covered entities," and that the intent of the Rule is not "to limit the level of security that may be agreed to between trading partners or others above this floor."[7] The authors of the preamble later state that "this final rule requires a floor of protection of all electronic health information. A covered entity has the option to exceed this floor. The sensitivity of information, the risks to and vulnerabilities

---

[6] FISMA (P.L. 107-347, Dec. 2002) requires each federal agency to develop, document, and implement an agency-wide program to provide information security for the information and information systems that support the operations and assets of the agency, including those provided or managed by another agency, contractor, or other source.

[7] Health Insurance Reform: Security Standards; Final Rule ("The HIPAA Security Rule"), 68 Fed. Reg. 34, 8334, 8345 (February 20, 2003). (incorporated at 45 CFR Parts 160, 162, and 164).

of electronic health information, and the means that should be employed to protect it are business determinations and decisions to be made by each covered entity."[8]

5.1 Health Insurance Portability and Accountability Act (HIPAA)

The Health Insurance Portability and Accountability Act of 1996 (HIPAA, Public Law 104-191) is the most well-known and influential law affecting the security and privacy practices of many healthcare organizations in the United States, specifically those that are "covered entities" under the Act. HIPAA will therefore affect the Capstone Policies of a great many of the expected participants in HIEs in the United States.

HIPAA required the Secretary of Health and Human Services (HHS) to create sets of regulations on several topics related to electronic healthcare transactions, including the privacy of health information (health information) and the security of electronic health information (ehealth information). Any private and secure health information exchange must therefore be able to support the standards of both the HIPAA Privacy Rule[9] and the HIPAA Security Rule.[10] This publication reflects the standards and implementation specifications of the HIPAA Security Rule that will drive the architectural framework and technical solutions of a mature HIE. However, the requirements of the Security Rule that do not necessarily create parameters or other requirements for the electronic exchange of health information are not explored. These requirements include policies and practices that may be implemented and enforced entirely at individual organizations, and are not relevant to the technical aspects of system interconnections. For a fuller discussion of the HIPAA Security Rule, including resources for understanding and addressing its requirements, see NIST Special Publication (SP) 800-66, Revision 1 (October 2008), *An Introductory Resource Guide for Implementing the Health Insurance Portability and Accountability Act (HIPAA) Security Rule*. For a discussion on the HIPAA Privacy Rule, see materials available through the HHS Office of Civil Rights at http://www.hhs.gov/ocr/privacy/hipaa/understanding/index.html.

5.2 Other Key Drivers for Capstone Policies

Other laws and regulations may also drive requirements for the functionality of security controls, depending on an HIE or its components' functions, activities, business partners, the types of information it handles, status as a government agency or private commercial entity, or even the identity of the legal jurisdiction in which it operates. This publication identifies many of the most common federal laws and regulations that create requirements for Capstone Policies for large numbers of organizations across the United States. However, not all relevant federal, state, and local laws and regulations are identified. In particular, this document does not identify the many state and local laws that may impact technology selection and implementation.

Table 1 lists a selection of the laws and regulations that may affect the healthcare transactions for some entities.

---

[8] The HIPAA Security Rule, 68 Fed. Reg. 34, 8355.
[9] Standards for Privacy of Individually Identifiable Health Information, Final Rule ("The HIPAA Privacy Rule"),
    65 Fed. Reg. 250, 82462 (incorporated at 45 CFR Parts 160, 162, and 164).
[10] 68 Fed. Reg. 34, 8334 (incorporated at 45 CFR Parts 160, 162, and 164).

Table 1. Capstone Policy Drivers and Their Implications

Capstone Policy Drivers	Entities Affected	Enabling Services Affected	Comment
American Recovery and Reinvestment Act of 2009, Public Law 111-5 (ARRA)	HIPAA-covered entities and their business associates; PHR vendors; and possibly other health-related organizations	Risk Assessment; Secured Communication Channel; Document Confidentiality	Requires the Office of the National Coordinator to establish two panels on health IT; holds business associates of HIPAA-covered entities directly responsible for certain standards of the Privacy and Security Rules; requires certain HIPAA covered entities to notify individuals who have been affected by breaches of their health information.
Federal Regulations: Initial Set of Standards, Implementation Specifications, and Certification Criteria for Electronic Health Record Technology, 45 CFR Part 170 (Interim Final Rule)	Eligible professionals and eligible hospitals under the Medicare and Medicaid EHR Incentive Programs	Risk Assessment; Secured Communication Channel; Document Confidentiality; Manage Consent Directives	The interim final rule became effective February 12, 2010. It adopts an initial set of standards, implementation specifications, and certification criteria, as required by section 3004(b)(1) of the Public Health Service Act. It represents the first step in an incremental approach to adopting standards, implementation specifications, and certification criteria to enhance the interoperability, functionality, utility, and security of health information technology and to support its meaningful use.
Federal Regulations: Protection of Human Subjects, 45 CFR Part 46 ("The Common Rule" for Human Subjects Protection)	Any institution conducting research involving human subjects conducted, supported, or otherwise subject to regulation by any federal department or agency	Risk Assessment; Document Confidentiality; Manage Consent Directives; De-Identification	Requires consent of research subjects, subject to some exemptions, including research on records where if the information is recorded by the investigator in such a manner that subjects cannot be identified, directly or through identifiers linked to the subjects. Consent forms must include notice of adequate provisions to protect the privacy of subjects and to maintain the confidentiality of data.
Federal Regulations: Protection of Human Subjects, 21 CFR Part 50 ("The FDA Rule" for Human Subjects Protection)	All institutions conducting clinical investigations regulated by the Food and Drug Administration or supporting applications for research or marketing permits for products regulated by the Food and Drug Administration.	Risk Assessment; Document Confidentiality; Manage Consent Directives	Requires consent of research subjects, subject to some exemptions, especially for research conducted on investigative new drugs (INDs). Consent forms must include notice of adequate provisions to protect the privacy of subjects and to maintain the confidentiality of data.

Capstone Policy Drivers	Entities Affected	Enabling Services Affected	Comment
Federal Regulations: Electronic Records; Electronic Signatures; Electronic Submissions; Establishment of Public Docket; Notice 28 CFR Part 11	Research facilities that transmit information to the Food and Drug Administration	Entity Identity Assertion (Authentication). Collect and Communicate Audit Trail; Document Integrity; Secured Communication Channel; Non-Repudiation of Origin	Especially relevant to transmission of information related to new drug trials.
Federal Regulations: Confidentiality of Alcohol and Drug Abuse Patient Records 42 CFR Part 2	Organizations that disclose patient alcohol and drug abuse records	Manage Consent Directives; Document Confidentiality	Restrictions on disclosing patient alcohol and drug abuse records. Intended to encourage patients to seek help for abuse and addiction.
Requirements Applicable to Programs for the Protection and Advocacy for Individuals with Mental Illness 42 CFR Part 51	Programs for the Protection and Advocacy for Individuals with Mental Illness ("P&A Programs") under Part C of the Developmental Disabilities Assistance and Bill of Rights Act (42 U.S.C. 6041, 6042)	Manage Consent Directives; Document Confidentiality	Restrictions on disclosing records concerning individuals who receive benefits from a P&A program, individuals that provide "general information or technical assistance on a particular matter," or individuals that report abuse or neglect.
Family Education Rights and Privacy Act of 2000 (FERPA) 20 U.S.C. § 1232g; 34 CFR Part 99	Public and private postsecondary educational institutions receiving federal funds	Manage Consent Directives; Document Confidentiality	FERPA protects education records of students enrolled at covered institutions. Its effect on health records is complex, but in general, health records are deemed to be "education records" if held by the covered institution.
Federal Medicaid Confidentiality Standards 42 CFR §431.300 et seq.	Medicaid providers	Manage Consent Directives; Document Confidentiality	Requires state Medicaid agencies to document rules for specifying the conditions for release and use of information about applicants and recipients.
Privacy Act of 1974 5 U.S.C. § 552a	Federal agencies and contractors	Manage Consent Directives; Document Integrity; Document Confidentiality; Risk Assessment	Requirements related to the collection, disclosure, and documentation of most personal information, including health information, held by federal agencies.

Capstone Policy Drivers	Entities Affected	Enabling Services Affected	Comment
Federal Information Security Management Act (FISMA) 44 U.S.C. § 3541	Federal agencies and contractors	Entity Identity Assertion (Authentication); Access Control (Authorization); Collect and Communicate Audit Trail; Document Integrity; Secured Communication Channel; Document Confidentiality; Non-Repudiation of Origin; Risk Assessment; Credential Management; Privilege Management	Among many other requirements, federal agencies must provide quarterly Privacy Management Report on privacy protections.
OMB Memoranda	Federal agencies and contractors	All	Various requirements related to privacy in the system development life cycle, analysis, reporting, and risk reduction relevant to federal agencies.

6.0   Enabling Services - Layer 2

Enabling Services are those services required to implement Capstone Policies. These services are typically HIE "context-independent," meaning they will be necessary for all HIEs although the manner of their implementation may be different. For example, two HIEs providing "Access Control" services might have different implementation models for addressing them.

The function of Enabling Services is to provide a standard set of minimum requirements across HIEs, but not to establish definitive methods for obtaining them. This means that every HIE will need to deploy Enabling Services using appropriate solutions that must be identified and selected. Having a consistent, standards-based set of Enabling Services can benefit future interoperability among HIEs. This standardization provides a basic assurance level on the implementation of security and privacy controls, and it will be easier to determine and address discrepancies among HIEs.

Services presented in this publication are derived from the Health Information Technology Standards Panel (HITSP) (www.hitsp.org) Security, Privacy, and Infrastructure constructs, which detail the selection of standards to meet the use case requirements, and common established security principles. These are then distilled to specifically address HIE data protection requirements. HIEs may identify other enabling services necessary to implement Capstone Policies through laws, regulations, policies, use cases, and other sources not specifically identified in this publication.

Figure 3. Enabling Services

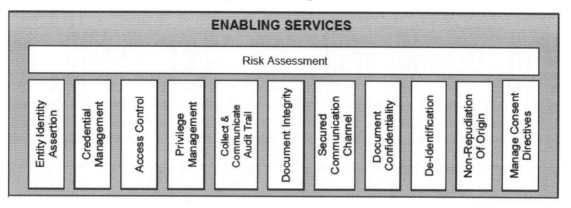

Table 2. Enabling Services and Definitions

Service Name	Source	Definition
Risk Assessment	Security and Privacy Principles	To identify security and privacy risks to HIE operations based on threats, assets, vulnerabilities, and likelihood of threat success.
Entity Identity Assertion (Authentication)	HITSP Construct	To ensure that an entity is the person or application that claims the identity provided.
Credential Management	Security Principles	To manage the life cycle of entity credentials used for authentication and authorization.
Access Control (Authorization)	HITSP Construct	To ensure that an entity can access protected resources if they are permitted to do so.
Privilege Management	Security Principles	To manage the life cycle of an entity's authorization attributes (e.g., roles, permissions, rules) for making access control decisions.
Collect and Communicate Audit Trail	HITSP Construct	To define and identify security-relevant events and the data to be collected and communicated as determined by policy, regulation, or risk analysis.
Document Integrity	HITSP Construct	To validate that the contents of a document have not been changed in an unauthorized or inappropriate manner.
Secured Communication Channel	HITSP Construct	To ensure that the mechanism through which information is shared or transmitted appropriately protects the authenticity, integrity, and confidentiality of transactions to preserve mutual trust between communicating parties.
Document Confidentiality	Security Principles	To prevent the unauthorized disclosure of a document that is exchanged or shared.
De-identification	Privacy Principles	To remove individual identifiers from a health record, or replace them with other information such as pseudonyms, so that it cannot be used to identify an individual.
Non-Repudiation of Origin	HITSP Construct	To provide the proof of the integrity and origin of data in an unforgeable relationship which can be verified by any party.
Manage Consent Directives	HITSP Construct	To ensure that individually identifiable health information is accessed only with an individual's consent.

6.1 Assumptions

Enabling Services identified in this section focus on the "exchange" aspect of HIE operations. To truly create a secure HIE environment, additional services are required to protect the data of the participating entities' organizational infrastructure (that is, the end points that house the data at rest). Some services exist to secure a participating entity's infrastructure, but only its internal infrastructure and activities. These services are not covered within the scope of this document. Many of the managerial and operational security controls that are not directly part of a cross-organization exchange of health information are also not addressed, but these measures may be critical for a complete security program for an organization. Organizations must ensure that these controls implemented in their HIEs are integrated and mutually supportive of the technology architecture derived from the design process outlined in this publication.

6.2 Enabling Services

The twelve Enabling Services identified below are derived from the HITSP Security, Privacy, and Infrastructure construct definitions and common established security principles. Information is provided, where available, to consolidate work previously conducted in this area in order to support a standardized, common vocabulary for HIE concepts.

In the following section, a definition and an illustrating example are provided for each service. Also provided is a list of other documents with further information regarding the specific enabling service. These referenced documents offer information for further insight and clarification.

6.2.1 Risk Assessment

Definition: To measure security and privacy risks to HIE operations that may adversely affect health information resulting in compromises of confidentiality (authorized information access and disclosure, including means for protecting personal privacy and proprietary information); integrity (guarding against improper information modification or destruction, including ensuring information non-repudiation of origin and authenticity), or availability (timely and reliable access to and use of information). Risk assessment, a component of risk management, incorporates threat and vulnerability analyses, the results of which may impact security architecture decisions.

Illustration: A county government decides to build an HIE to research heart disease. HIE-participating entities perform a comprehensive risk assessment by examining the information to be exchanged over the network. They decide to categorize the information into three assurance levels (low, medium, high) based on the sensitivity of the information. The community then decides what measures are required for each assurance level. Specific threats are evaluated for their potential to exploit existing vulnerabilities and documented as risks. Existing measures are evaluated for their ability to mitigate these risks, and additional measures are decided upon to ensure that residual risks are acceptable. The complete set of security controls is documented and used in a trust agreement enforced by the HIE governance body.

Other References:
HIPAA Security Rule: 45 CFR 164.308(a)(1), Implementation Specification: Risk Analysis.

NIST Publications:
- SP 800-30, *Risk Management Guide for Information Technology Systems.*
- Draft SP 800-39, *Managing Risk from Information Systems: An Organizational Perspective.*
- SP 800-53 Rev. 3, *Recommended Security Controls for Federal Information Systems and Organizations,* security control family: Risk Assessment (RA).

6.2.2 Entity Identity Assertion (Authentication)

Definition: To ensure that an entity is the person or application that claims the identity provided.

Illustration: Doctor at Hospital One wishes to access Patient's records for the purposes of entering new data concerning Patient's health status. This new data may later be accessed by other healthcare providers that are members of the HIE. Before accessing Patient's record, Doctor is asked to provide a username, a password, and a security token device to prove Doctor's identity. The enabling service then uses a predefined procedure, based on the sensitivity of the records Doctor is requesting, to authenticate Doctor.

Other References:

HITSP: C19, Entity Identity Assertion.

NHIN Core Service: Subject Discovery.

HIPAA Security Rule: 45 CFR 164.308(a)(5), Implementation Specification: Password Management; 45 CFR 164.312(a)(1), Implementation Specification: Unique User Identification; 45 CFR 164.312(d), Standard: Person or Entity Authentication.

NIST Publications:
- SP 800-53 Rev. 3, *Recommended Security Controls for Federal Information Systems and Organizations,* security control family: Identification and Authentication (IA).
- Draft SP 800-63 Rev. 1, *Electronic Authentication Guideline.*

6.2.3 Credential Management

Definition: To create and manage the life cycle of entity credentials (e.g., username/password, public and private keys, biometrics) used for authentication and access control.

Illustration: Hospital One has three assurance levels for the information exchanged on its network. For information of each assurance level, acceptable authentication credentials and the life cycle of those credentials are defined. The credential life cycle includes an identity proofing process to obtain, validate, renew, and revoke the credential.

Other References:

HIPAA Security Rule: 45 CFR 164.312(d), Standard: Person or Entity Authentication.

NIST Publications:
- SP 800-53 Rev. 3, *Recommended Security Controls for Federal Information Systems and Organizations,* security controls: AC-2, Account Management; IA-4, Identifier Management; IA-5, Authenticator Management.
- SP 800-57, *Part 1, Recommendation for Key Management - Part 1: General.*
- Draft SP 800-63 Rev. 1, *Electronic Authentication Guideline.*

6.2.4 Access Control (Authorization)

Definition: To ensure that an entity can access protected resources only if they are permitted to do so.

Illustration: Doctor at Hospital needs to access the information system supporting Hospital's participation in the HIE. After verifying Doctor's identity (Entity Identity Assertion), the system retrieves the access control policy and permissions associated with Doctor's identity to render a grant or deny decision.

Other References:

HITSP: TP20, Access Control; SC108, Access Control Service Collaboration.

NHIN Core Service: Authorization Framework, Consumer Preference Profile.

HIPAA Security Rule: 45 CFR 164.308(a)(4), Implementation Specification: Access Authorization, Implementation Specification: Access Establishment and Modification.

NIST Publications:

- SP 800-53 Rev. 3, *Recommended Security Controls for Federal Information Systems and Organizations,* security control family: Access Control (AC).

6.2.5 Privilege Management

Definition: To manage the life cycle of an entity's authorization attributes (e.g., roles, permissions, rules) for making access control decisions.

Illustration: Doctor from Hospital participates in an HIE that conducts research as well as provides clinical care. The Doctor has access to certain research projects within the network. The research HIE administrator assigns several roles to Doctor's account in the system to associate their identity with the research projects in which the Doctor is involved. Then, permissions are created for Doctor to access and use the information needed to participate in each research project. When any research project is changed or finished, the HIE administrator will update Doctor's role and permissions accordingly.

Other References:

NHIN Core Service: Authorization Framework, Consumer Preference Profile.

HIPAA Security Rule: 45 CFR 164.308(a)(4), Standard: Information Access Management.

NIST Publications:

- SP 800-53 Rev. 3, *Recommended Security Controls for Federal Information Systems and Organizations,* security controls: AC-2, Account Management; AU-6, Audit Review, Analysis, and Reporting.

6.2.6 Collecting and Communicating Audit Trails

Definition: To define and identify security-relevant events and the data to be collected and communicated as determined by policy, regulation, or risk analysis to support identification of those security-relevant events.

Illustration: System Administrator reviews a file that is generated by the HIE-enabling system on a daily basis. The Audit Trail enabling service generates a record of the users who have accessed what files and when. The enabling service also makes note of any attempts to access the system from an unauthorized terminal; the use of an expired username or password, unusual numbers of password attempts, and other potential attempted violations of security policies. The System Administrator may take appropriate action to ensure that future attempts at gaining unauthorized access are unsuccessful.

Other References:

HITSP: T15, Collect and Communicate Security Audit Trail; SC109, Security Audit Service Collaboration.

NHIN Core Service: Query Audit Log.

HIPAA Security Rule: 45 CFR 164.308(a)(5), Implementation Specification: Log-In Monitoring, 45 CFR 164.312(b), Standard: Audit Controls.

NIST Publications:

- SP 800-53 Rev. 3, *Recommended Security Controls for Federal Information Systems and Organizations,* security control family: Audit and Accountability (AU).
- SP 800-92, *Guide to Computer Security Log Management.*

6.2.7 Ensuring Document Integrity

Definition: To validate that the contents of a document have not been changed in an unauthorized or inappropriate manner.

Illustration: Hospital One sends a record to Hospital Two using a one-way hash to confirm that the record has not been altered in transit.

Other References:

HITSP: TP13, Manage Sharing of Documents.

HIPAA Security Rule: 45 CFR 164.308(a)(5), Implementation Specification: Protection from Malicious Software; 45 CFR 164.312(c)(1), Standard: Integrity; 164.312(e)(1), Implementation Specification: Integrity Controls.

NIST Publications:

- SP 800-25, *Federal Agency Use of Public Key Technology for Digital Signatures and Authentication.*
- SP 800-53 Rev. 3, *Recommended Security Controls for Federal Information Systems and Organizations,* security control family: System and Information Integrity (SI); security control: Transmission Integrity (SC-8).
- SP 800-106, *Randomized Hashing Digital Signature.*
- FIPS 186-3, *Digital Signature Standard (DSS)*

6.2.8 Secure Communication Channel

Definition: To ensure the authenticity, the integrity, and the confidentiality of transactions, and the mutual trust between communicating parties.

Illustration: Hospital One and Hospital Two are part of an HIE. When exchanging information, the communication channel is protected through various security and privacy controls to ensure that security and privacy requirements are met. For example, Transport Layer Security (TLS) is used to encrypt the channel, and patient consent information will be verified and exchanged before sending health information.

Other References:

HITSP: T17, Secured Communication Channel; TN907, Common Data Transport Technical Note.

NHIN Core Service: Messaging Platform.
HIPAA Security Rule: 45 CFR 164.312(e)(1), Standard: Transmission Security; Implementation Specification: Encryption.

NIST Publications:

- SP 800-45, Version 2, *Guidelines on Electronic Mail Security.*
- SP 800-52, *Guidelines for the Selection and Use of Transport Layer Security (TLS) Implementations.*
- SP 800-53 Rev. 3, *Recommended Security Controls for Federal Information Systems and Organizations,* security control family: System and Communications Protection (SC).
- SP 800-58, *Security Considerations for Voice Over IP Systems.*
- SP 800-77, *Guide to IPsec VPNs.*
- SP 800-113, *Guide to SSL VPNs.*

6.2.9   Preserving Document Confidentiality

Definition: To ensure that sensitive health information is not sent intentionally or unintentionally to a party that is not authorized to view it.

Illustration: Hospital One sends health records to Hospital Two. Hospital One sends the document using previously agreed-upon encryption methods to ensure the confidentiality of the exchanged health records.

Other References:

HITSP: TP13, Manage Sharing of Documents.

HIPAA Security Rule: 45 CFR 164.312(e)(1), Standard: Transmission Security; Implementation Specification: Encryption.

NIST Publications:

- Draft FIPS 140-3, *Security Requirements for Cryptographic Modules.*
- SP 800-45, Version 2, *Guidelines on Electronic Mail Security.*
- SP 800-52, *Guidelines for the Selection and Use of Transport Layer Security (TLS) Implementations.*
- SP 800-53 Rev. 3, *Recommended Security Controls for Federal Information Systems and Organizations,* security control family: System and Communications Protection (SC), Transmission Confidentiality (SC-9).
- SP 800-57, *Recommendation for Key Management*
- SP 800-58, *Security Considerations for Voice Over IP Systems.*
- SP 800-77, *Guide to IPsec VPNs.*
- SP 800-111, *Guide to Storage Encryption Technologies for End User Devices.*
- SP 800-113, *Guide to SSL VPNs.*

6.2.10 De-Identification

Definition: To ensure that individuals' records have all data elements removed before the data is shared for statistical, research, public health, or other reasons that do not benefit the data subject directly, and for which no authorization has been provided, such that there is no reasonable basis to believe that the information can be used to identify an individual. De-identification can be accomplished by removing the data permanently (anonymization); permanently replacing each data element removed with a placeholder, sometimes called a "token" (pseudonymization); or replacing each datum with a unique token and maintaining a record (usually through a third party) such that it is possible to re-identify the individual through appropriate channels, such as having a third party contact the individual's care provider (reversible pseudonymization, or re-identification).

Illustration: Researcher at Hospital wants to study the records of all patients with a particular form of cancer within a certain age range. The Researcher contacts their organization's research review board to confirm that the protocol will be conducted ethically and within all state, federal, and local laws and guidelines. The Researcher then contacts all providers in the HIE and asks them to help populate a database of de-identified information. Providers contact all patients fitting the profile and secure their consent. Each provider then uses the De-Identification enabling service to remove all potentially identifying information from each consenting patient's record, and then sends the record to Researcher. Thereafter, no further patient consent will be required to further share or disclose the de-identified data. Because ages are a relevant research parameter, birth years are retained in each record, although exact birth dates are removed.[11]

Other References:

HITSP: T24, Pseudonymize; C25, Anonymize; C87, Anonymize Public Health Case Reporting Data ; C88, Anonymize Immunizations and Response Management Data Component; C164, Anonymize Newborn Screening Data Component; C165, Anonymize Long Term and Post Acute Care Data Component.

NHIN Core Service: Authorized Case Follow-up.

HIPAA Privacy Rule references: The requirements for de-identification under the HIPAA Privacy Rule are explicitly laid out in Section 45 CFR 164.514, *Other requirements relating to uses and disclosures of health information*, subsections (a) (Standard: de-identification of health information), (b) (Implementation specifications: requirements for de-identification of health information), and (c) (Implementation specifications: re-identification).

NIST Publications:

- SP 800-122, *Guide to Protecting the Confidentiality of Personally Identifiable Information (PII)*.

6.2.11 Non-Repudiation of Origin

Definition: To provide proof of the integrity and the origin of data in a relationship that has not been forged, and which can be verified by any party.

---

[11] This illustration addresses several issues of potential varying interpretations by Institutional Review Boards and/or Privacy Boards. For example, some HIPAA analysts interpret the Privacy Rule that patient consent must be received to send patient information into a database or similar repository for the purposes of being de-identified. Where possible varying interpretations exist, the scenario adopts the most stringent requirements; it also intentionally avoids complications such as the availability of limited data sets.

Illustration: Patient transfers from Hospital One to Hospital Two. Hospital Two requests Hospital One to send Patient's health information. Hospital One dates and signs the record transfer using its private key and follows the non-repudiation of origin procedure agreed by both hospitals. After the record transfer, any entity who has access to Patient's record can verify that the record is indeed transferred from Hospital One.

Other References:

HITSP: C26, Nonrepudiation of Origin.

HIPAA Security Rule: 45 CFR 164.312(d), Standard: Person or entity authentication.

NIST Publications:

- SP 800-25, *Federal Agency Use of Public Key Technology for Digital Signatures and Authentication.*
- SP 800-53 Rev. 3, *Recommended Security Controls for Federal Information Systems and Organizations,* security control: Non-Repudiation (AU-10).

6.2.12 Managing Consent Directives

Definition: To ensure that health information is collected, accessed, used, or disclosed only with a consumer's consent.

Illustration: Hospital and Specialist are both entities within the same HIE. Hospital sends Patient's health information to Specialist. Specialist will review the health information and provide a medical opinion, but will not interact with Patient directly. Specialist's own in-house rules require that Hospital confirms that Patient has signed an authorization for a specific clinical trial. The Managing Consent Directives service would enable Specialist to confirm that Patient has consented to the specific clinical trial, provided authorization for data use, and authorization for organizational access. Additionally, any changes to prior privacy policies (such as when a patient changes their level of participation or requests that data no longer be made available) have been recorded.

Later, Specialist wishes to de-identify Patient's data and share it with Researcher, also an HIE participant. Under HIPAA, patients must provide adequate consent before their data is sent to a repository for de-identification, so Specialist asks Hospital to contact Patient to provide the necessary consent. Patient provides the consent, and when it is reflected via the enabling service, the Specialist de-identifies the record and submits it to Researcher's repository.

Other References:

HITSP: TP30, Manage Consent Directives; CAP143, Manage Consumer Preference and Consents.

NHIN Core Service: Consumer Preferences Profile.

HIPAA Privacy Rule: See Subpart E generally, especially 45 CFR 164.506, Consent for uses or disclosures to carry out treatment, payment, and healthcare operations.

7.0   Enabling Processes – Layer 3

The Enabling Processes define business processes for Enabling Services. While Enabling Services are a nomenclature for an HIE's data protection requirements, Enabling Processes expand the Enabling Services into detailed requirements, usually in the forms of use cases or scenarios, based on an HIE's business practices. Enabling Processes are HIE context-dependent (see discussion of "context" in Section 3.0). Hence, HIEs of different contexts could implement the same Enabling Services with different Enabling Processes. The following paragraph is an example of Enabling Processes for an "Access Control" service:

Joan Taylor owns a protein database at a research institution. Her protein database is used in the *Hope research project* HIE with research scientists from a local university. Joan defines the following processes for the "Access Control" service:

- Only the Hope research project manager has read/write privileges to the database. However, the project manager can delegate read/write privileges to research project members.

- The database will be open for Hope research project use from 10:00 a.m. to 3:00 p.m. every day. Joan wants to reserve the other time slots for the research institution scientists.

- All accesses, internal and external, to the protein database need to be logged.

As illustrated in this example, enabling processes are the detailed requirements for enabling services. They are written in plain English and are derived from an HIE participant's business practices. Enabling processes should be clearly defined for each enabling service, and fully vetted within the HIE context.

8.0   Notional Architecture – Layer 4

Capstone Policies (Layer 1), Enabling Services (Layer 2), and Enabling Processes (Layer 3) serve as the inputs to create the Notional Architecture, which will guide subsequent selections and decisions about technical solutions. The Notional Architecture defines major architecture constructs and their relationships to the implementation of Enabling Processes. It is standards-based and technology- and vendor-neutral. The Notional Architecture is dependent on the Enabling Processes and will vary between HIE implementations. In addition to the inputs from the Capstone Policies, Enabling Services, and Enabling Processes, the Notional Architecture must consider *architecture design principles*, guiding principles derived from the experiences of organizations that have implemented information sharing networks, and *architecture constructs*, design structures that can serve as the basic building blocks for a Notional Architecture.

The Notional Architecture development process is illustrated in Figure 4.

Figure 4. Notional Architecture Development Process

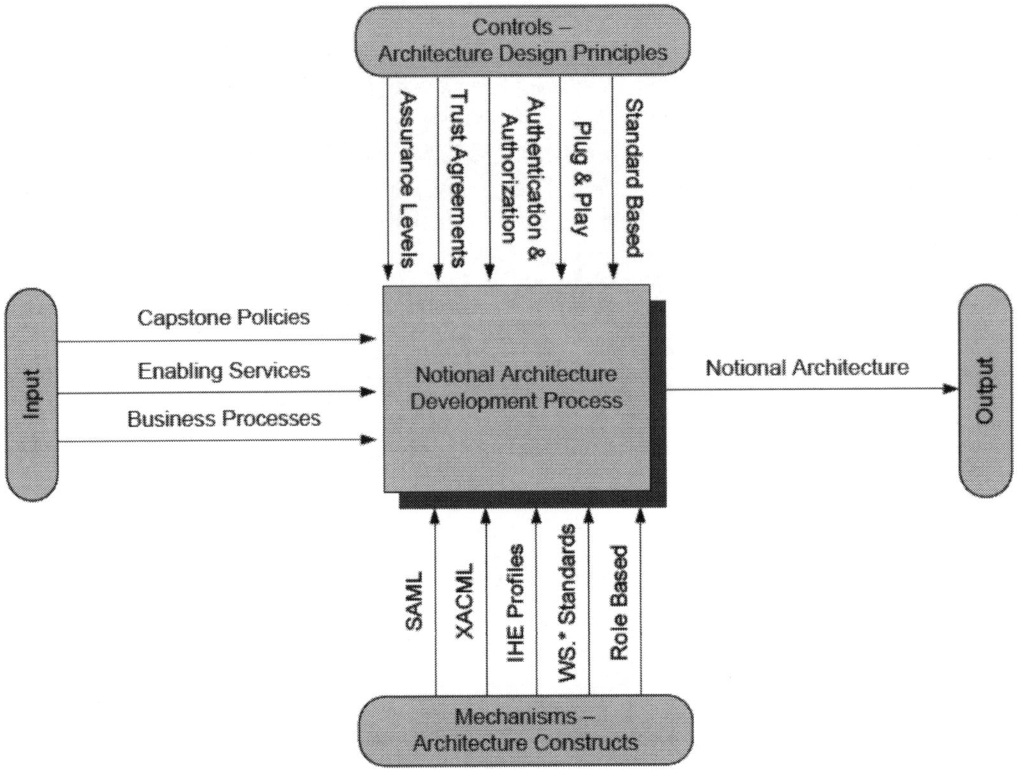

8.1 Architecture Design Principles

Architecture design principles are best practices derived from large-scale information-sharing implementations. Design principles serve as the overall guidance for building security and privacy services for HIEs. This publication identifies five design principles. These principles suggest that system designers take the following actions to ensure that their resulting architectures are as robust as possible. System designers should:

- Conduct a risk assessment to determine appropriate assurance levels for shared information;

- Create a "master" trust agreement describing requirements for a trust domain (trust domain is defined in Section 8.1.2);

- Separate authentication/credential management and authorization/privilege management;

- Develop data protection capabilities as plug-and-play services; and

- Maintain a standards-based, technology-neutral, and vendor-neutral architecture.

These design principles are described in more detail in the following sections.

8.1.1 Conduct a Risk Assessment to Determine Appropriate Assurance Levels for Shared Information

Conducting a risk assessment on the information exchanged in any HIE is fundamental and critical to the effective protection of the information. Organizations should be aware of the security and privacy risks with the exchanged information in order to design a proper architecture.

The results of a risk assessment can enable HIE transactions to be categorized into assurance levels. Assurance levels define the degree of confidence required to conduct a specific HIE transaction. The assurance levels reflect the sensitivity and criticality of the information. The following table lists several examples of HIE transactions with associated assurance levels.

Table 3. Illustrative Examples of Assurance Levels

Assurance level (Relative)	Example HIE Transactions	Information Classification
Low	Share aggregate data on quality and outcomes	Public information
Medium	Share patient demographic health information	Sensitive information
High	Share patient HIV information	Confidential information

Assurance levels are represented by a range (e.g., 1-2-3; high-medium-low, gold-silver-bronze) rather than absolute values due to their comparative nature. The representation of assurance levels helps an organization decide what kind of credential and what identity-proofing process is needed for each type of transaction (see Section 8.1.3 for details on assurance levels and authentication credentials). The number of required assurance levels depends on the complexity of the information exchanged among participants in the HIE.

8.1.2 Create a "Master" Trust Agreement Describing Security and Privacy Requirements for a Trust Domain

Once assurance levels are defined and risks are identified and mitigated, a trust domain can be created. A trust domain is a logical construct within which a single set of access control policies can be enforced for all transactions conducted between HIE participants. An enforceable master trust agreement will provide all HIE participants a basic level of assurance and avoids the complexity of creating individual trust agreements between every two entities. The master trust agreement should be honored in every HIE transaction. For unique HIE transactions, specialized trust agreements might be created based on the master trust agreement. At a minimum, if the trust agreement is not honored, participants have some recourse for appropriately allocating responsibility for resulting harms.

8.1.3 Separate Authentication/Credential Management and Authorization/Privilege Management

Authentication is the process of verifying an entity's identity using authentication credentials. Authorization is the process of deciding whether an authenticated entity can execute a specific function or access certain information using authorization attributes.

Credential management governs the types of authentication credentials and their life cycle based on defined assurance levels. Table 4 lists examples of credentials of various assurance levels specific to credential management.

Table 4. Authentication Assurance Levels are Mapped to Authentication Credentials

Assurance level	Authentication Credentials and Required Processes
Level 1 – Low	PIN # or password
Level 2 – Medium	Strong password, one-time password / ID proof
Level 3 – High	PKI credential / ID proof
Level 4 – Very High	Hard crypto token / ID proof

Credential management grants an entity its identity within the HIE context. The identity usually has a global effect within a specific HIE. Once an HIE credential is granted to an entity, it will be recognized across the HIE context until it is revoked or expired.

Privilege management governs the privileges of an HIE entity (i.e., what an entity will be allowed to do once it has been authenticated). Granting privileges requires a trusted credential for an HIE entity who requests access to certain information. The decision to grant privileges is usually made locally by the HIE entity which guards the requested information.

Authentication, Credential Management, Authorization, Privilege Management, and Storage are basic components of identity and access management illustrated in Figure 5.

Figure 5. Basic Identity and Access Management Components

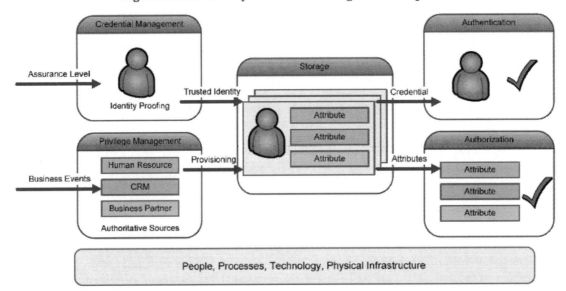

The concepts of authentication/credential management and authorization/privilege management (global authentication vs. local authorization) are related but highly distinguishable, and therefore these two topics should be separated when an organization is developing its Notional Architecture. The trust agreement should identify what kinds of credentials will be accepted for authorization at each assurance level in an HIE. HIE entities which guard requested information need to use an interoperable authorization language to express authorization policies, including but not limited to roles, rules, and permissions. In most cases, depending on the requirements, authorization decisions will need to be made locally at HIE entities such that HIE entities which guard the information will assume full authority on granting access privileges.

The creation of a trust agreement can be made easier when credential management and privilege management are separated. Having the global authentication credential and local authorization authority allows HIE entities to better control what information is exposed to HIEs and what information should be protected inside their own boundaries.

8.1.4 Develop Data Protection Capabilities as Plug-and-Play Services

As described under "Enabling Services," the word "services" refers to the protections that a requester should be able to expect in each information exchange, regardless of whether the requester explicitly and knowingly makes such a request for these protections. Modeling data protection capabilities as services will have the following benefits:

- *Plug-and-play:* Service users do not need to know the implementation details and interoperability is improved;

- *Loose coupling:* Plug-and-play services are loosely coupled so they are scalable as requirements change;

- *Efficiency:* Instead of having every entity create its own services, the entities can use a common set of services; and

- *Effectiveness:* It is easier to enforce if every transaction goes through the same set of services.

Developing data protection capabilities as services also improves future interoperability with other HIEs.

8.1.5 Maintain a Standards-Based, Technology-Neutral, and Vendor-Neutral Architecture

Standards-based, technology-neutral, and vendor-neutral characteristics are important for a Notional Architecture. These characteristics will aid in driving the selection of technical solutions and standards while maintaining forward compatibility as the solutions landscape evolves.

8.2 Architecture Constructs

Architecture constructs, usually originating from various industry standards, identify basic building blocks for a Notional Architecture. This section lists several important architecture constructs only as illustrative examples.

8.2.1 Security Assertion Markup Language (SAML)

SAML, developed by the Security Services Technical Committee of the Organization for the Advancement of Structured Information Standards (OASIS), is an Extensible Markup Language (XML)-based framework for communicating user authentication, entitlement, and attribute information. SAML allows business entities to make assertions regarding the identity, attributes, and entitlements of a subject (an entity that is often a human user) to other entities, such as a partner company or another enterprise application. SAML is a flexible and extensible protocol designed to be used – and customized if necessary – by other standards.

For more information on SAML, visit www.oasis-open.org.

8.2.2 eXtensible Access Control Markup Language (XACML)

XACML was ratified as an OASIS standard in February 2003 (1.0 version). XACML defines a generic authorization architecture and the constructs for expressing and exchanging access control policy information using XML. Policy constructs include policies, rules, combining algorithms, etc. XACML complements SAML so that policy decisions, as well as the policies themselves, can be exchanged in a standard fashion.

For more information on XACML, visit www.oasis-open.org.

8.2.3 Integrating the Healthcare Enterprise (IHE) Profiles

IHE is a global initiative that creates the framework for passing vital health information seamlessly – from application to application, system to system, and setting to setting – across multiple healthcare enterprises. IHE brings together health information technology stakeholders to implement standards for communicating health information efficiently throughout and among healthcare enterprises by developing a framework for interoperability.

For more information on IHE profiles, visit www.ihe.net.

8.2.4 Web Services Security Standards

Web services security standards represent various specifications defined to implement Web services security. Figure 6 identifies Web services security standards.

Figure 6. Web Services Security Standards

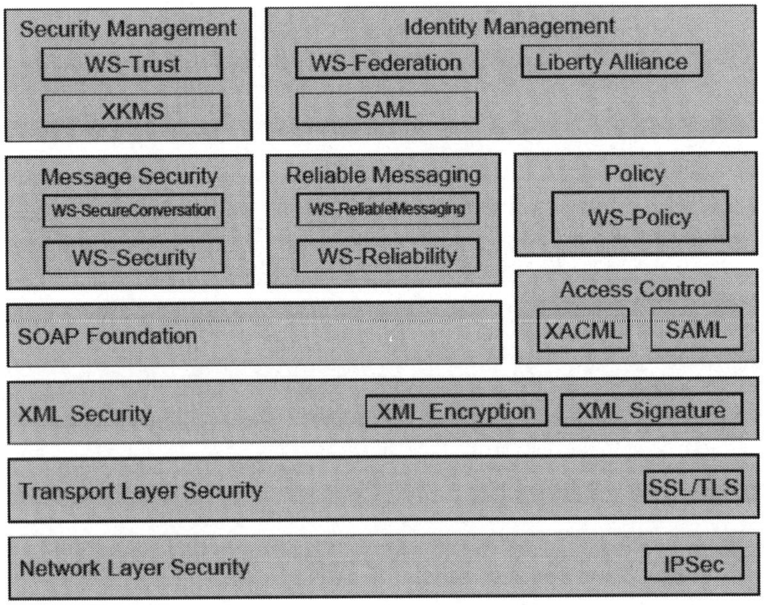

Web services security standards are composable standards. Depending on the Notional Architecture, an implementation might use only one or two standards from the entire Web services security stack.

For more information on Web services security, visit www.oasis-open.org.

8.2.5 Role-Based Access Control (RBAC)

With role-based access control, access decisions are based on the roles that individual users have as part of an organization. Users take on assigned roles (e.g., doctor, nurse, billing specialist, office manager). Access rights are grouped by role name, and the use of resources is restricted to individuals authorized to assume the associated role. For example, within a hospital system, the role of doctor can include operations to perform diagnoses, prescribe medications, and order laboratory tests, and the role of researcher can be limited to gathering anonymous clinical information for studies.

For more information on RBAC, visit http://csrc.nist.gov/groups/SNS/rbac/.

8.2.6 Attribute-Based Access Control (ABAC)

An attribute-based access control model recognizes that a flexible access control policy should address the evaluation of multiple dimensions of an entity, including identifiers, roles, and qualifications. Since roles can be viewed as nothing more than attributes of principals, RBAC can be wholly absorbed into an attribute-based mechanism.

Attribute-based authorization policies have some distinct advantages over other approaches. First, an attribute-based approach recognizes from its inception that a flexible access control policy cannot be locked into evaluating only one dimension of a principle (such as an identity or role). For example, in order to provide proper controls for accessing health information, it may be necessary to consider various other principal attributes such as doctor qualifications, formal access approvals, or organization affiliation. Second, an attribute-based approach takes into consideration that there are other attributes that are relevant to authorization policies besides those associated with resources or environmental attributes.

9.0 Technology Solutions and Standards – Layer 5

Once the Notional Architecture is complete, the final layer is to select the technical solutions and data standards that will satisfy the requirements for secure and private services of the architecture. The following figure shows illustrative steps taking an organization from a Notional Architecture to the implementation of secure HIE services.

Figure 7. Illustrative Steps from Notional Architecture to Secure HIE Services

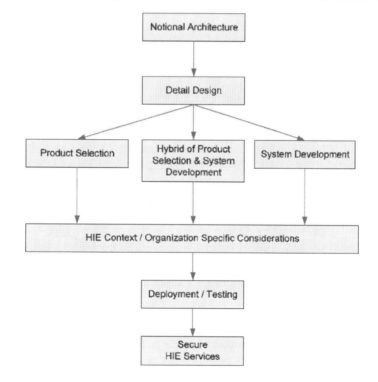

While a Notional Architecture defines architecture constructs and their relationships, the detailed design transforms a Notional Architecture into detailed implementation specifications that are ready for product selection, system development, or a hybrid of the two. In taking this final step, many HIE contexts and organization-specific considerations will need to be evaluated. For example, if most of the HIE participants use Java development resources, Java-related technical solutions might be a better choice than others. Once technical solutions and data standards are selected, they must be deployed and tested to verify that HIE services are truly private and secure.

10.0   Building a Nationwide HIE using Regional HIEs

As discussed in Section 3, this publication presents a five-layer operating model for building security architectures for Regional HIEs. If Regional HIEs follow the five-layer operating model, there will be many Regional HIEs using a standard set of data protection services, as illustrated in Figure 8.

Figure 8. Regional HIEs with Standard Enabling Services

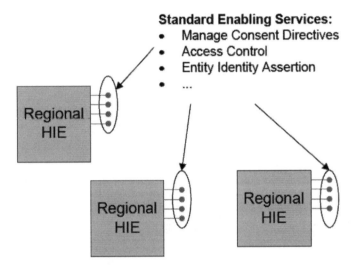

Although it is likely that each Regional HIE might implement the services differently based on its own HIE requirements, having a standard set of services allows for a common understanding of assurance levels that can allow for risk-based interconnection decisions. For example, while HIEs might have different access control policies and implementations, the existence of a common, shared access control service provides a foundation from which to further evaluate risk.

Using Regional HIEs as the building blocks, Multi-Regional HIEs can be built using a federated architecture as illustrated in Figure 9. The federated architecture will centralize certain elements (e.g., trust agreements, assurance levels) while allowing the Regional HIE to remain autonomous.

Figure 9. Multi-Regional HIE with Federated Enabling Services

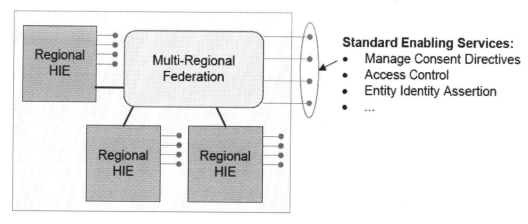

A Nationwide HIE can be constructed in a similar way by connecting Multi-Regional HIEs using a federated architecture as illustrated in Figure 10.

Figure 10. Nationwide HIE with Federated Data Protection Services

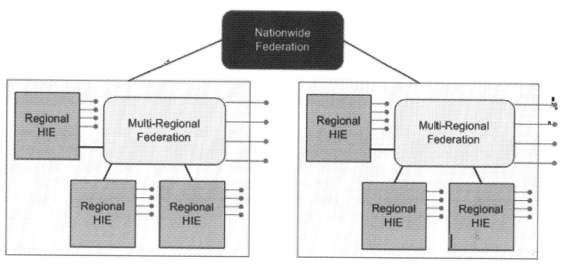

This publication provides a standardized systematic design methodology for developing a security architecture and technical solutions that support a core set of Enabling Services necessary for the secure exchange of health information. The overarching premise is that if entities engaged in the exchange of health information use a standard approach for the selection of security architectures, the ability to scale these HIEs into larger constructs will be dramatically increased.

In this appendix, the security architecture design process is applied to a specific American Health Information Community (AHIC) use case to illustrate the analyses and considerations that need to be made when applying this process to the exchange of health information. This scenario considers issues and data flows surrounding the implementation of information technology to enable the delivery of personalized healthcare. This case is supplied for illustrative purposes only, and may not consider all the complexities, requirements, and interdependencies that could be encountered in particular environments. No changes or alterations were made to the AHIC use case, and the functionalities and uses of the technologies may well differ from those of current and future HIEs.

The use case was developed in two stages. First, a "Prototype Use Case" was developed, which described the data flows of the use case at a high level. AHIC solicited public feedback on the Prototype Use Case in February 2008. Feedback was received and incorporated into the "Detailed Use Case," which comprehensively documents all of the events and actions within the use case at a detailed level.

Figure 11. Clinical Assessment Scenario of 2008 ONC Personalized Healthcare Use Case

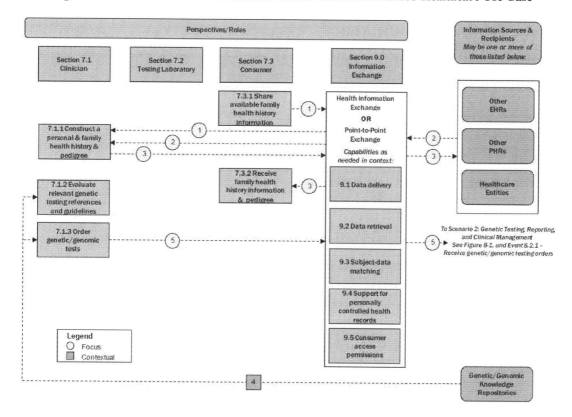

The detailed Personalized Healthcare use case was further broken out into two scenarios. This document uses the Clinical Assessment scenario[12] to describe how the implementation of the security architecture design process would affect it. Data protection issues are analyzed at each

---

[12] For detailed definitions of each perspective, role, and action in the Clinical Assessment scenario, please refer to the 2008 ONC Personalized Healthcare use case: http://www.hhs.gov/healthit/usecases/phc.html.

layer of the operating model. Only one enabling service, however, is further defined in subsequent layers in this document.

A.1 Illustrative Clinical Assessment Scenario

Carol uses a publicly available Web-based Personal Health Record (PHR) system to store her personal medical history, including health conditions of her parents and her genetically related relatives. Carol then begins seeing Dr. Alice, and grants her access to read her PHR.

With Carol's authorization, Dr. Alice retrieves Carol's PHR from the Web-based system. To make a sound clinical assessment, Dr. Alice asks for Carol's permission to request additional information from her previous family doctor, Dr. Bob. She also asks Carol for more information on the health conditions and health history of her parents and for "read and write" permissions in order to make appropriate entries in Carol's PHR. Having received Carol's authorization, Dr. Alice obtains the information and constructs a consolidated view of Carol's personal and family health history. While reviewing Carol's health records, Dr. Alice finds several duplications and consolidates them in Carol's PHR.

Dr. Alice uses the consolidated information to conduct a clinical assessment and develop a diagnostic plan. With Carol's authorization, Dr. Alice incorporates new inputs into Carol's PHR system.

A.2 Identifying the Health Information Exchanges

Figure 12 provides a graphical representation of the exchanges of health information that occur in this illustrative clinical assessment scenario.

Figure 12. Illustrative Clinical Assessment Scenario

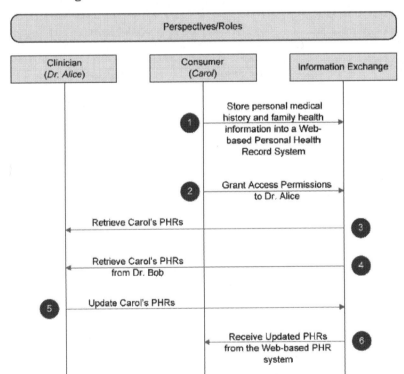

The six exchanges of health information are:

1. Carol stores personal medical history and family health information into a Web-based Personal Health Record (PHR) system;
2. Carol grants access permissions to Dr. Alice;
3. Dr. Alice retrieves Carol's personal medical history and family health information from the Web-based PHR;
4. Dr. Alice retrieves Carol's personal medical information from her previous doctor, Dr. Bob;
5. Dr. Alice incorporates new inputs into Carol's PHR; and
6. Carol, at her request, receives a copy of her updated PHR.

The HIE security architecture design methodology will be applied to this scenario to demonstrate how it enables the secure exchange of health information.

A.3 Identifying Capstone Policies – Layer 1

Capstone Policies include the federal, state, and local laws and regulations, and organizational policies that apply to the exchange of health information in this illustrative example.

A.3.1 Federal Laws and Regulations

The most significant data protection requirements governing the exchange described are the HIPAA Privacy and Security Rules (as modified by the HITECH Act of ARRA). Other federal laws and regulations may govern other kinds of healthcare transactions, particularly those that involve exchanges of health information with particular government agencies; healthcare research activities; exchanges of particularly sensitive health information (such as information about substance abuse treatment); or sharing health information for purposes other than healthcare treatment, payment, or operations (such as law enforcement, public health reporting, or marketing). Given this scenario, however, HIPAA is certainly the most significant driver of a relevant Capstone Policy, although others will also be applicable.

A.3.2 State and Local Laws and Regulations

Depending on the state and jurisdiction, other rules may govern the use, disclosure, or security of health information. For example, a majority of states require entities conducting business in the state to provide notice to all affected individuals in the event of a breach or loss of private data, including health information.

In cases where state law conflicts with HIPAA, HIPAA explicitly allows state law to take precedence over HIPAA if the state law is "more stringent." That is, the state law supplies even greater protections to an individual's privacy or requires additional or stronger security protections than those required by HIPAA.

In the current case, it is assumed that relevant state law:

- Requires the disclosure of health information to any healthcare provider at the patient's written request. HIPAA merely allows covered entities to share health information with other healthcare providers for payment, treatment, or operations purposes. As disclosure is compelled under this hypothetical state law, it is "more stringent" and must be followed.

- Forbids the disclosure of health information to a patient's otherwise authorized representative if, in the judgment of the healthcare provider, releasing that information could cause the patient harm. Many states have a provision like this one such that healthcare providers would not, for example, be obliged to disclose health information about mental or physical abuse to the patient's possible abuser. As this measure allows the patient even more protection than HIPAA explicitly allows, it is "more stringent" and should be followed.

- Requires the provider to disclose to the patient or a patient's representative or guardian if there is a known or suspected breach of the patient's unencrypted information.

A.3.3 Organizational Policies

Further requirements may be imposed by the institutions at which Dr. Alice and Dr. Bob practice. While HIPAA sets parameters for data protection, its standards often require the institution to implement their own policies, appropriate to their individual institutions' sizes, resources, and risk profiles. Other individual institutional rules may be driven by other laws, such as the Common Rule for Human Subjects Research, institutional accreditation standards, contractual obligations with business partners, or best practices.

This scenario assumes that certain appropriate rules apply to the Web-based PHR system used by Carol. Rules will be proposed only to the extent necessary to address one enabling service, Entity Identity Assertion. These rules are not intended to be complete, and no assertion is made as to their adequacy for any real-world entity or environment.

This scenario assumes that the following institutional rules apply for Carol's access to her PHR:

- Carol, and anyone to whom she grants access to her account, must log in using a unique username and password.

- Passwords must have a minimum "strength" as defined in organizational policy.

- Carol, and anyone to whom she grants access to her account, must use a digital certificate to access her account.

- Carol, and anyone to whom she grants access to her account, must use a hardware token to assert their identity.

- Carol has unrestricted access to her own PHR.

- Carol has unlimited privileges to grant access and privileges to others, including privileges to read, write, edit, or delete her account.

In addition, other institutional-level restrictions may apply to Dr. Alice's and Dr. Bob's institutions. Dr. Alice and Dr. Bob may have to log on to their accounts using separate identity assertion controls.

A.4 Identify Enabling Services - Layer 2

The operating model identified the twelve Enabling Services that every HIE should consider. Based on the six identified HIE activities (as illustrated in Figure 12), the following table lists Enabling Services that should be used in each HIE:

Table 5. Enabling Services for Each HIE

HIE #	HIE Description	Enabling Services	Enabling Services Description
1	Carol stores her and her family's	Risk Assessment	Risk assessment is used to analyze the business risks of compromising the security and privacy of the health information exchanged.

HIE #	HIE Description	Enabling Services	Enabling Services Description
	health information into a Web-based Personal Health Record (PHR) system.	Entity Identity Assertion	The Web-based PHR requires Carol to identify herself using a registered credential every time she logs in.
		Access Control	The Web-based PHR grants access permissions based on privileges an authenticated individual has.
		Credential Management	The Web-based PHR that Carol selects will require Carol to use certain types of credentials to register.
		Privilege Management	Carol has full access permissions to her PHR, and she can assign access permissions to her doctors.
		Audit Trail	All accesses to Carol's Web-based PHR will be logged. Suspicious accesses will trigger warning messages that will be sent to Carol.
		Secure Communication Channel	All information transmitted is secured between Carol's terminal and the Web-based PHR.
2	Carol grants access permissions to Dr. Alice.	Entity Identity Assertion	The Web-based PHR requires Carol to identify herself using registered credentials every time she logs in.
		Access Control	The Web-based PHR allows Carol to change access permissions associated with her PHR.
		Privilege Management	Carol assigns access permissions on certain portions of her personal medical history to Dr. Alice.
		Audit Trail	The Web-based PHR maintains a record of Carol's action of assigning access permissions to Dr. Alice.
		Secure Communication Channel	All information transmitted is secured between Dr. Alice's terminal and the Web-based PHR.
3	Dr. Alice retrieves Carol's health information from the Web-based PHR.	Entity Identity Assertion	The Web-based PHR requires Dr. Alice to identify herself with a registered credential.
		Access Control	The Web-based PHR allows Dr. Alice to read the portion of Carol's PHR to which she has access permission.
		Audit Trail	Dr. Alice's access to Carol's PHR is logged.
		Secure Communication Channel	All information transmitted is secured between Carol's terminal and the Web-based PHR.
4	Dr. Alice retrieves Carol's health information from Dr. Bob.	Entity Identity Assertion	Dr. Bob requires Dr. Alice to identify herself with registered credentials. Dr. Alice requires Dr. Bob to identify himself with registered credentials.
		Manage Consent Directives	Dr. Bob obtains Carol's consent to share Carol's personal medical information.
		Secure Communication Channel	All information transmitted is secured between Dr. Alice and Dr. Bob.
	Dr. Alice	Entity Identity Assertion	The Web-based PHR requires Dr. Alice to identify herself with registered credentials.

HIE #	HIE Description	Enabling Services	Enabling Services Description
5	incorporates new inputs into Carol's PHR.	Access Control	The Web-based PHR allows Dr. Alice to read and append Carol's PHR to which she has access permission.
		Audit Trail	Dr. Alice's access to Carol's PHR is logged.
		Secure Communication Channel	All information transmitted is secured between Dr. Alice's terminal and the Web-based PHR.
6	Carol receives an update from her PHR system.	Entity Identity Assertion	The Web-based PHR requires Carol to identify herself using registered credentials every time she logs in.
		Access Control	The Web-based PHR allows Carol to read her personal medical history.
		Audit Trail	Carol's access to her PHR will be logged.
		Secure Communication Channel	All information transmitted is secured between Carol's terminal and the Web-based PHR.

The identified Enabling Services need to be in place to enable the exchange activities among Dr. Alice, Carol, Dr. Bob, and the Web-based PHR system. Implementation of one enabling service, Entity Identity Assertion, is addressed in the following sections.

A.5 Develop Enabling Processes – Layer 3

The Entity Identity Assertion service of the Web-based PHR system has the following requirements based on the exchange activities indicated in the illustrative scenario above.

- The system shall accept three types of credentials to authenticate users (including service providers, consumers, and any others):
  - o User-created ID with strong password;
  - o Digital certificates; and
  - o Hardware tokens.

- The system shall authenticate every transaction.

- The system shall accept credentials (any of the three types) issued from trusted third parties.

A.5.1 Authentication Credentials

The system has defined the following processes on how three types of credentials can be accepted:

Table 6. Processes for Credential Acceptance

Credentials	Processes
User ID and Password	• User ID must be unique. • Passwords must be stored in irreversible encrypted form, and the password file cannot be viewed in unencrypted form. • A password must not be displayed on the data entry/display device. • Passwords must be at least eight characters long. • Passwords must be composed of at least three of the following: English uppercase letters, English lowercase letters, numeric characters, and special characters. • Password lifetime will not exceed 60 days.

Credentials	Processes
	• Users cannot use the previous six passwords. • The system will give the user a choice of alternative passwords from which to choose. • Passwords must be changed by the user after initial logon.
Digital Certificates	• The certificate must be an X.509v3 certificate. • The certificate must be within the valid period. • The certificate must be verified and validated through authentication. • The system will not issue digital certificates. Users will present trusted third party-issued certificates that are valid and verifiable by the system.
Hardware Tokens	• The system will accept and support preapproved types of hardware tokens as authentication credentials.

A.5.2 Accepting Trusted Third-Party-Issued Credentials

The system defines its processes and policies of accepting third-party authentication credentials as follows:

Table 7. Acceptance of Third-Party Authentication Credentials

Credentials	Processes
User ID and Password	• A trusted third party must comply with the system's User ID and Password rules (e.g., minimum password strength requirements must be met). • The system shall accept authentication claims from a third-party authentication authority. • The third-party authentication claim shall comply with the system's profile for authentication claims.
Digital Certificates	• Since the system will not issue digital certificates, all certificates will be issued by trusted third parties. • The system shall only accept digital certificates issued by authorities that comply with the system's X.509 profile. • The system's X.509 profile defines requirements to be a trusted certificate authority and the certificate validation process.
Hardware Tokens	• User can only request hardware tokens from the system. No third-party hardware tokens will be accepted.

As illustrated above, the Enabling Processes further refine the Entity Identity Assertion service for the Web-based PHR system. The Enabling Processes will vary for different exchange activities. These processes will translate into part of the governance policies which could be part of the trust agreement between HIE entities.

A.6 Develop Notional Architecture – Layer 4

Based on the defined Enabling Processes, a Notional Architecture can be developed for the Entity Identity Assertion service. This Notional Architecture is a standards-based, platform-independent, and vendor-neutral implementation blueprint for Enabling Services and Processes, and it will drive the selection of technical solutions.

Figure 13 provides an illustrative example of the Notional Architecture for the Web-based PHR system's Entity Identity Assertion Service.

Figure 13. Illustrative Notional Architecture for Entity Identity Assertion Service

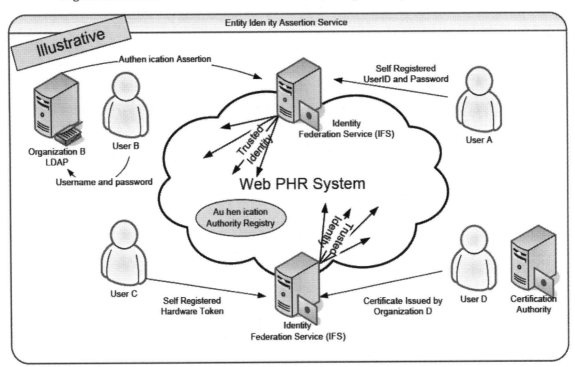

In the Notional Architecture, four different scenarios are described:

- Self-Registered UserID and Password (User A): Users register themselves with the Web-based PHR system by creating a User ID and password. Users must go through the identity-proofing process defined by the Web-based PHR system.

- Third-Party UserID and Password (User B): Users are redirected to their home organizations to perform the authentication. The home organization's (Organization B) authentication authority (e.g., LDAP) will issue a SAML assertion to the Web-based PHR system as the authentication credential.

- Hardware Token (User C): Users who request hardware tokens from the Web-based PHR system can use the issued token as the authentication credential.

- Third-Party Certificates (User D): Users use third-party issued certificates as authentication credentials.

The Identity Federation Service (IFS) will serve as the authentication portal which accepts all types of credentials and creates a trusted identity for authenticated users into the Web-based PHR system. The trusted identity could be a digital certificate or a SAML assertion.

A.7 Select Technical Solutions – Layer 5

Once the Notional Architecture is determined, technical solutions can be selected and deployed to implement the architecture. An illustrative example of the deployment of possible technical solutions is depicted in Figure 14.

Figure 14. Illustrative Technical Solutions for Entity Identity Assertion Service

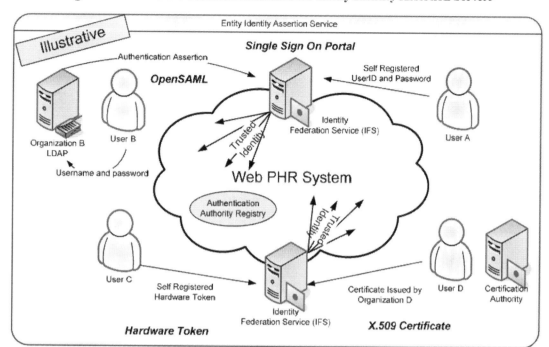

A.8 Considerations for Health Information Exchanges

Following a similar process as illustrated above, an organization can implement all Enabling Services necessary to facilitate the secure and private exchange of health information in this scenario. The services described in this architecture design methodology focus only on the exchange portion. They do not focus on those services necessary to implement security and privacy protections for data used solely within the involved organizations. To provide end-to-end protection of health information, the involved organizations need to implement relevant services that provide adequate protection for the information outside the bounds of exchange.

The actual data exchange--that is, the act of transmitting and receiving the health information--is a point of particular vulnerability to the security and privacy of consumer information in the health information exchange because it is usually done outside of the participating organizations' security boundaries. However, to ensure that a consumer's health information is adequately protected, the "non-exchange" portions of the data usage, including collection, storage, modification, and destruction, must also receive security and privacy protections, which may include disaster recovery and contingency planning, configuration management, and other processes and technologies.

Appendix B: Acronyms

ABAC	Attribute-Based Access Control
AC	Access Control (NIST SP 800-53 Security Control Family)
AHIC	American Health Information Community
ARRA	American Recovery and Reinvestment Act
AU	Audit and Accountability (NIST SP 800-53 Security Control Family)
CSRC	Computer Security Resource Center
FISMA	Federal Information Security Management Act
EHR	Electronic Health Record
FIPS	Federal Information Processing Standard
HHS	Health and Human Services
HIE	Health Information Exchange
HIPAA	Health Insurance Portability and Accountability Act
HIT	Health Information Technology
HITECH	Health Information Technology for Economic and Clinical Health
HITSP	Healthcare Information Technology Standards Panel
IA	Identification and Authentication (NIST SP 800-53 Security Control Family)
ID	Identity
IHE	Integrating the Healthcare Enterprise
IPsec	Internet Protocol Security
IT	Information Technology
LDAP	Lightweight Directory Access Protocol
MOU	Memorandum of Understanding
NeHC	National eHealth Collaborative
NHIN	Nationwide Health Information Network
NIST	National Institute of Standards and Technology
NISTIR	National Institute of Standards and Technology Interagency Report
NOPP	Notice of Privacy Practices
OASIS	Organization for the Advancement of Structured Information Standards
ONC	Office of the National Coordinator
PHR	Personal Health Record
PIN	Personal Identification Number
PKI	Public Key Infrastructure
RA	Risk Assessment (NIST SP 800-53 Security Control Family)
RBAC	Role-Based Access Control
SAML	Security Assertion Markup Language
SC	Systems and Communications (NIST SP 800-53 Security Control Family)
SI	System and Information Integrity (NIST SP 800-53 Security Control Family)
SLA	Service-Level Agreement

SP	Special Publication
SSL	Secure Socket Layer
TLS	Transport Layer Security
USB	Universal Serial Bus
VPN	Virtual Private Network
WS	Web Services
XACML	Extensible Access Control Markup Language
XML	Extensible Markup Language

Appendix C: Glossary

Terms	Definitions
Access Control (Authorization)	To ensure that an entity can only access protected resources if they have the appropriate permissions based on the predefined access control policies.
Ad Hoc HIEs	An Ad Hoc HIE occurs when two healthcare organizations exchange health information, usually under the precondition of familiarity and trust, using existing and usual office infrastructure such as mail, fax, e-mail and phone calls.
Architecture Constructs	Design structures that can serve as the basic building blocks for a Notional Architecture.
Architecture Design Principles	Best practices derived from large-scale information-sharing implementations that serve as the overall guidance for building security and privacy services for HIEs.
Availability 44 U.S.C., Sec. 3542	Ensuring timely and reliable access to and use of information.
Capstone Policies	Those policies that are developed by governing or coordinating institutions of HIEs. They provide overall requirements and guidance for protecting health information within those HIEs. Capstone Policies must address the requirements imposed by: (1) all laws, regulations, and guidelines at the federal, state, and local levels; (2) business needs; and (3) policies at the institutional and HIE levels.
Collecting and Communicating Audit Trails	To define and identify security-relevant events and the data to be collected and communicated as determined by policy, regulation, or risk analysis to support identification of those security-relevant events.
Confidentiality 44 U.S.C., Sec. 3542	Preserving authorized restrictions on information access and disclosure, including means for protecting personal privacy and proprietary information.
Credential	A set of attributes that uniquely identifies a system entity such as a person, an organization, a service, or a device.
Credential Management	To manage the life cycle of entity credentials used for authentication.

Terms	Definitions
De-Identification	To ensure that individuals' records have all data elements removed before the data is shared for statistical, research, public health, or other reasons that do not benefit the data subject directly, and for which no authorization has been provided, such that there is no reasonable basis to believe that the information can be used to identify an individual. De-identification can be accomplished by removing the data permanently (anonymization); permanently replacing each data element removed with a placeholder, sometimes called a "token" (pseudonymization); or replacing each datum with a unique token and maintaining a record (usually through a third party) such that it is possible to re-identify the individual through appropriate channels, such as having a third party contact the individual's care provider (reversible pseudonymization, or re-identification).
Enabling Processes	Define the operational baseline via use cases and scenarios for Enabling Services. Enabling Processes are HIE context-dependent. Two HIEs could, for example, have different Enabling Processes implementing the same Enabling Service (e.g., "Access Control").
Enabling Services	Define the nomenclature of services required to implement Capstone Policies. Enabling Services are designed to be HIE context-independent. Services presented in this publication are derived from common industry-wide data protection practices and then customized to specifically address the requirements of HIEs.
Ensuring Document Integrity	To validate that the content of a document has not been changed in an unauthorized or inappropriate manner.
Entity Identity Assertion (Authentication)	To ensure that an entity is the person or application that claims the identity provided.
Hardware Token	A physical object that is used to provide strong authentication of the holder's identity. A common hardware token is a smart card that is swiped or scanned. Other types include small devices with digital displays of constantly shifting login information or USB keys that must be plugged into devices' ports before they can be used to prove one entity's identification.
Health Information Exchange (HIE)	A health information organization that brings together healthcare stakeholders within a defined geographic area and governs health information exchange among them for the purpose of improving health and care in that community.
Integrity 44 U.S.C., Sec. 3542	Guarding against improper information modification or destruction, and includes ensuring information non-repudiation and authenticity.
Managing Consent Directives	To ensure that individually identifiable health information is collected, accessed, used, or disclosed only with a consumer's consent.

Terms	Definitions
Multi-Regional HIEs	Multi-Regional HIEs connect multiple Regional HIEs. They may cross state lines or other physical boundaries. They are usually EHR-based. Since they connect multiple Regional HIEs, they will likely have a federated technical architecture.
Nationwide HIEs	A Nationwide HIE would connect many Regional or Multi-Regional HIEs. It would require the use of some form of EHR, involve multiple state jurisdictions, and have a nationwide federated technical architecture.
Non-repudiation	To ensure that information received can be confirmed as having been sent by the apparent sender and that no reasonable basis exists for claiming that the information came from some other source; and to ensure that the sender can confirm that the intended recipient has received the information.
Notional Architecture	Defines the technical constructs (e.g., role-based access control and directory services) and their relationships to implement Enabling Processes. Notional Architecture is the blueprint to drive the selection of technical solutions and data standards. Notional Architecture is standards-based, technology-neutral, and vendor-neutral.
Preserving Document Confidentiality	To ensure that personal health information is not sent intentionally or unintentionally to a party that is not authorized to view it, either by the patient or by a provider that has received the patient's authorization or a waiver of the patient's authorization.
Privilege	One entity's permissions to access information and to execute functions.
Privilege Management	To manage users' permissions (whether those permissions are granted or denied) to access information or to execute functions associated with entities for HIE transactions.
Regional HIEs	Those that consist of two or more legally and commercially independent institutions that share EHRs, but where no state jurisdictional issues exist that prevent or impede the sharing of data.
Risk Assessment	To identify risks to HIE operations that may compromise protected health information resulting in compromises of confidentiality (authorized information access and disclosure, including means for protecting personal privacy and proprietary information); integrity (guarding against improper information modification or destruction, including ensuring information non-repudiation and authenticity), or availability (timely and reliable access to and use of information).
Secure Communication Channel	To ensure that the mechanism through which information is shared or transmitted is subject to minimized risks to the authenticity, integrity, and confidentiality of transactions to preserve mutual trust between communicating parties.

Appendix D: References

Public Laws

Public Law 104-191, Health Insurance Portability and Accountability Act (HIPAA) of 1996, August 21, 1996.

Public Law 107-347, E-Government Act of 2002 (Title III: Federal Information Security Management Act [FISMA] of 2002), December 17, 2002.

Public Law 111-5, American Recovery and Reinvestment Act of 2009 (ARRA) (Title XIII, Health Information Technology for Economic and Clinical Health [HITECH] Act of 2009), February 17, 2009.

Federal Regulations

Health Insurance Reform: Security Standards; Final Rule ("The HIPAA Security Rule"), 68 FR 8334, February 20, 2003 (incorporated at 45 CFR Parts 160, 162, and 164).

Standards for Privacy of Individually Identifiable Health Information, Final Rule ("The HIPAA Privacy Rule"), 65 Fed. Reg. 250, 82462, December 28, 2000 (incorporated at 45 CFR Parts 160 and 164).

Standards for Privacy of Individually Identifiable Health Information; Final Rule (modifications to the HIPAA Privacy Rule), 67 Fed. Reg. 157, 53181, August 14, 2002 (incorporated at 45 CFR Parts 160 and 164).

Federal Information Processing Standards (FIPS) Publications

FIPS 140-3, *Draft Security Requirements for Cryptographic Modules*, July 2007.

FIPS 186-3, *Digital Signature Standard (DSS)*, June 2009

NIST Special Publications (SPs)

NIST SP 800-25, *Federal Agency Use of Public Key Technology for Digital Signatures and Authentication*, October 2000.

NIST SP 800-30, *Risk Management Guide for Information Technology Systems*, January 2002.

NIST SP 800-39, *Draft Managing Risk from Information Systems: An Organizational Perspective*, April 2008.

NIST SP 800-45, Version 2, *Guidelines on Electronic Mail Security*, February 2007.

NIST SP 800-52, *Guidelines for the Selection and Use of Transport Layer Security (TLS) Implementations*, June 2005.

NIST SP 800-53, Revision 3, *Recommended Security Controls for Federal Information Systems and Organizations*, August 2009.

NIST SP 800-57, *Recommendation for Key Management*, March 2007.

NIST SP 800-58, *Security Considerations for Voice Over IP Systems*, January 2005.

NIST SP 800-63 Rev. 1, *Draft Electronic Authentication Guide*, December 2008.

NIST SP 800-66, Revision 1, *An Introductory Resource Guide for Implementing the Health Insurance Portability and Accountability Act (HIPAA) Security Rule*, October 2008.

NIST SP 800-77, *Guide to IPsec VPNs*, December 2005.

NIST SP 800-92, *Guide to Computer Security Log Management*, September 2006.

NIST SP 800-106, *Randomized Hashing Digital Signatures*, July 2008.

NIST SP 800-111, *Guide to Storage Encryption Technologies for End User Devices*, November 2007.

NIST SP 800-113, *Guide to SSL VPNs*, July 2008.

NIST SP 800-122, *Guide to Protecting the Confidentiality of Personally Identifiable Information (PII)*, April 2010.

Web Sites and Other Resources

Department of Health and Human Services (DHHS): www.hhs.gov

Healthcare Information Technology Standards Panel (HITSP): www.hitsp.org

NIST Computer Security Resource Center (CSRC): http://csrc.nist.gov/

Office of the National Coordinator for Health Information Technology (ONC): healthit.hhs.gov

65282712R10031

Made in the USA
Lexington, KY
08 July 2017